The Complete KETO Beverage Recipe Book For Women

Delicious And Keto-Friendly Drinks To Stay In Shape

Megan Kelly

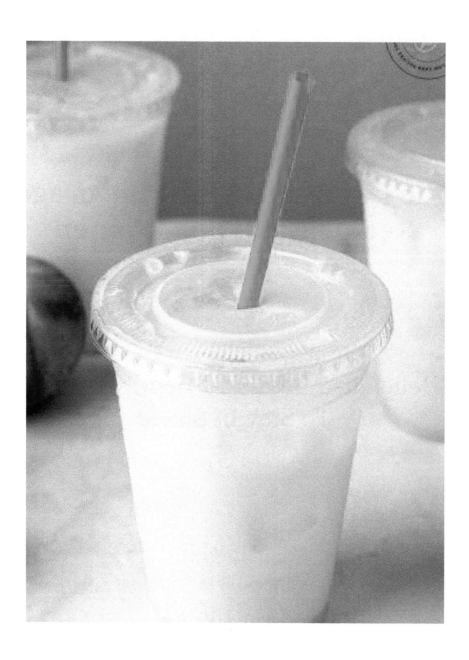

Table of contents

6

Coffee With Cream

Servings: 1

Time: 5 mins

Difficulty: Easy

Nutrients per serving: Calories: 203 kcal | Fat: 21g | Carbohydrates: 2g | Protein: 2g | Fiber: 0g

Ingredients

- 1/4 Cup Heavy Whipping Cream
- 2 Tbsps. Nuts, Crushed (Optional)
- 3/4 Cup Brewed Coffee

Method

1. Brew your coffee according to your preference.
2. Slightly heat the cream in a pan and stir till it becomes frothy.
3. Take a cup and mix the warm cream and coffee in it.
4. Serve hot with crushed nuts on top or as it is.

Keto Coffee

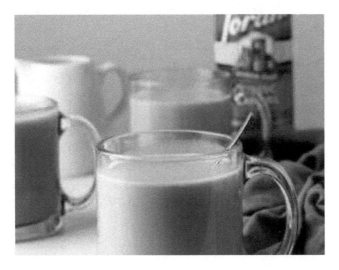

Servings: 2

Time: 5 mins

Difficulty: Easy

Nutrients per serving: Calories: 260 kcal | Fat: 27.7g | Carbohydrates: 1.05g | Protein: 1.08g | Fiber: 0g

Ingredients

- 2 Tbsps. Coconut Oil Or MCT Oil
- 2 Tbsps. Butter, Unsalted (Grass-Fed)

- 2 Cups Brewed Coffee
- 1 Tsp. Vanilla Extract (Optional)
- 1 Tbsp. Heavy Whipping Cream (Optional)

Method

1. Brew your coffee according to your preference.
2. Blend the coffee with unsalted butter, coconut or MCT oil, vanilla extract, and whipping cream if you want, in a blender for about a minute or until it becomes frothy.
3. Pour out the keto coffee in your favorite mugs and enjoy.

Vegan Keto Golden Milk

Servings: 1

Time: 5 mins

Difficulty: Easy

Nutrients per serving: Calories: 303 kcal | Fat: 31.1g | Carbohydrates: 2.7g | Protein: 2.1g | Fiber: 2g

Ingredients

- 2 Tsps. Ginger, Fresh & Peeled
- 2 Tbsps. MCT Oil
- 1 & 1/2 Cup Almond Milk, Unsweetened
- 2 Tsps. Erythritol
- 1/4 Tsp. Cinnamon, Ground
- 2 Ice Cubes
- 3/4 Tsp. Turmeric Powder
- 1/4 Tsp. Vanilla Extract
- Sea Salt, To Taste

Method

1. Combine all the ingredients in a blender and mix for about a quarter or half a minute.
2. For the strong taste of turmeric and ginger, blend longer.
3. Decant into the glass or mug and sprinkle powdered cinnamon on top before serving.

Keto Creamy Chocolate Smoothie

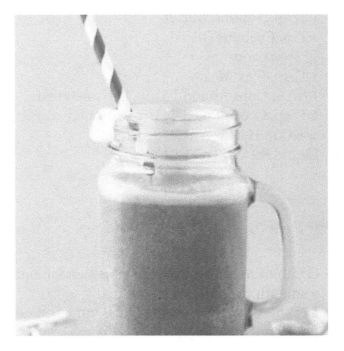

Servings: 2

Time: 10 mins

Difficulty: Easy

Nutrients per serving: Calories: 593.3 kcal | Fat: 55.7g | Carbohydrates: 7.7g | Protein: 10.6g | Fiber: 11.7g

Ingredients

- 1 Tbsp. Almond Butter
- 1 Tsp. Coconut Oil
- 1/2 Avocado
- 1 Tbsp. Flax Meal
- 1 & 1/4 Cups Almond Milk, Unsweetened
- 1 Tbsp. Cocoa Powder, Unsweetened
- 1/4 Cup Heavy Whipping Cream
- Liquid Stevia, To Taste

Method

1. Combine all the ingredients in a blender and mix until a smooth consistency is attained.
2. Decant into the serving glass and top with cocoa powdered and whipped cream if you want.

Keto Pumpkin Pie Spice Latte

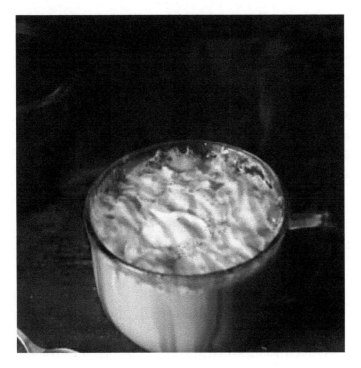

Servings: 3

Time: 10 mins

Difficulty: Easy

Nutrients per serving: Calories: 136.28 kcal | Fat: 19.83g | Carbohydrates: 2.49g | Protein: 0.68g | Fiber: 1.79g

Ingredients

- 2 Tbsps. Butter
- 1/2 Tsp. Cinnamon, Powdered
- 1 Cup Coconut Milk
- 2 Cups Brewed Coffee
- 2 Tsps. Pumpkin Pie Spice
- 1/4 Cup Pumpkin Puree
- 1 Tsp. Vanilla Extract
- 2 Tbsps. Heavy Whipping Cream
- 15 Drops Liquid Stevia

Method

1. Pour the coconut milk, butter, pumpkin puree, and spices into a small saucepan and heat over a medium-low flame.
2. Once the mixture starts to bubble, add the coffee, and mix well.
3. Remove from the heat and add the whipped cream and liquid Stevia. Mix well to blend the contents until frothy.
4. Decant in the serving mug and a dollop of whipped cream on top.

Blueberry Banana Bread Smoothie

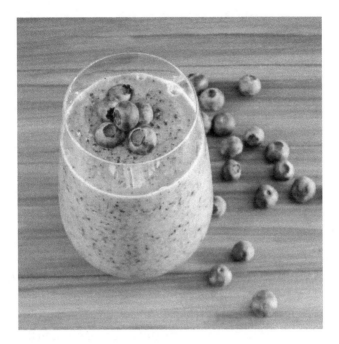

Servings: 2

Time: 10 mins

Difficulty: Easy

Nutrients per serving: Calories: 270 kcal | Fat: 23.31g | Carbohydrates: 4.66g | Protein: 3.13g | Fiber: 5.65 g

Ingredients

- 1/4 Cup Blueberries
- 2 Tbsps. MCT Oil
- 2 1 & 1/2 Tsps. Banana Extract
- Cups Vanilla Coconut Milk, Unsweetened
- 1 Tbsp. Chia Seeds
- 3 Tbsps. Golden Flaxseed Meal
- 10 Drop Liquid Stevia
- 1/4 Tsp. Xanthan Gum

Method

1. Combine all the ingredients in a blender and let it sit for a few minutes to allow the chia and flax seeds to soak some moisture.
2. Then blend for a minute or two until a smooth consistency is attained.
3. Serve in the glasses and enjoy.

Blackberry Chocolate Shake

Servings: 2

Time: 5 mins

Difficulty: Easy

Nutrients per serving: Calories: 346 kcal | Fat: 34.17g | Carbohydrates: 4.8g | Protein: 2.62g | Fiber: 7.4g

Ingredients

- 1/4 Cup Blackberries
- 2 Tbsps. MCT Oil
- 1 Cup Coconut Milk, Unsweetened
- 1/4 Tsp. Xanthan Gum
- 2 Tbsps. Cocoa Powder
- 12 Drops Liquid Stevia
- 7 Ice Cubes

Method

1. Combine all the ingredients in a blender and blend for a minute or two until a smooth consistency is attained.
2. Serve in the glasses and enjoy.

Dairy-Free Dark Chocolate Shake

Servings: 2

Time: 5 mins

Difficulty: Easy

Nutrients per serving: Calories: 349.35 kcal | Fat: 33.15g | Carbohydrates: 5.73g | Protein: 7.2g | Fiber: 6.1g

Ingredients

- 1/2 Avocado
- 1/2 Cup Coconut Cream, Chilled
- 2 Tbsps. Hulled Hemp Seeds
- 2 Tbsps. Dark Chocolate (Low Carb)
- 1/2 Cup Almond Milk
- 1 Tbsp. Cocoa Powder
- 2 Tbsps. Powdered Erythritol, To Taste
- Flake Salt, To Taste
- 1 Cup Ice

Method

1. Put the cocoa powder, hemp seeds, erythritol, and dark chocolate in a blender and mix until the chocolate is chopped.
2. Add the remaining ingredients and blend for a minute or two until a smooth consistency is attained.
3. Pour in the serving glasses and enjoy.

Keto Meal Replacement Shake

Servings: 2

Time: 5 mins

Difficulty: Easy

Nutrients per serving: Calories: 453 kcal | Fat: 42.6g | Carbohydrates: 6.9g | Protein: 8.8g | Fiber: 8.1g

Ingredients

- 1/2 Avocado
- 2 Tbsps. Almond Butter
- 1 Cup Almond Or Coconut Milk, Unsweetened
- 1/4 Tsp. Vanilla Extract
- 1/2 Tsp. Cinnamon, Powdered
- 2 Tbsps. Golden Flaxseed Meal
- 1/8 Tsp. Salt
- 2 Tbsp. Cocoa Powder
- 1/2 Cup Heavy Cream
- 15 Drops Liquid Stevia
- 8 Ice Cubes

Method

1. Combine all the ingredients in a blender and blend for a minute or two until a smooth consistency is attained.
2. Serve in the glasses and enjoy.

Keto Iced Coffee

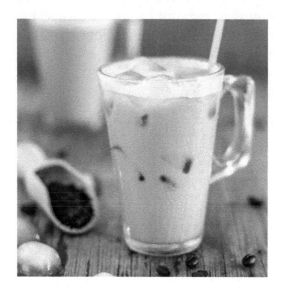

Servings: 1

Time: 5 mins

Difficulty: Easy

Nutrients per serving: Calories: 160 kcal | Fat: 16.1g | Carbohydrates: 1.5g | Protein: 1.6g | Fiber: 0g

Ingredients

- 3 Tbsps. Heavy Cream

- 5 Drops Liquid Stevia
- 1 Cup Brewed Coffee
- 1/2 Tsp. Vanilla Extract (Optional)
- Ice Cubes, To Taste

Method

1. Brew your coffee according to your preference and let it cool down to room temperature.
2. Combine the coffee with all the other ingredients in a blender and blend for about a minute or until it becomes frothy.
3. Pour the iced coffee in your favorite mug and enjoy.

Low-Carb Ginger Smoothie

Servings: 2

Time: 5 mins

Difficulty: Easy

Nutrients per serving: Calories: 83 kcal | Fat: 8g | Carbohydrates: 3g | Protein: 1g | Fiber: 1g

Ingredients

- 2 Tbsps. Spinach, Frozen
- 1/3 Cup Coconut Milk Or Cream, Unsweetened
- 2 Tsps. Ginger, Fresh & Grated
- 2 Tbsps. Lime Juice, Divided
- 2/3 Cup Water

For Garnishing
- 1/2 Tsp. Fresh Ginger, Grated

Method

1. Combine all the ingredients in a blender and adjust the lime juice amount as per your taste.
2. Blend the mixture for a minute or until a smooth consistency is attained.
3. Serve with grated ginger on top.

Whipped Dairy-Free Low-Carb Dalgona Coffee

Servings: 2

Time: 5 mins

Difficulty: Easy

Nutrients per serving: Calories: 40 kcal | Fat: 2g | Carbohydrates: 1g | Protein: 1g | Fiber: 1g

Ingredients

- 2 Tbsps. Water, Hot
- 1 & 1/2 Cups Coconut Or Almond Milk, Unsweetened
- 1 & 1/2 Tbsps. Erythritol
- 1 & 1/2 Tbsps. Espresso Instant Coffee Powder
- 1/2 Cup Ice Cubes
- 1 Tsp. Vanilla Extract (Optional)

Method

1. Take a narrow glass and combine the coffee powder, hot water, and erythritol in it and blend them well with

an immersion blender for about 3 minutes or till the mixture becomes creamy and light in color.

2. Take two glasses, fill two-third of them with ice and then pour the almond or coconut milk in it along with vanilla extract if you want. Mix them well.

3. Put the spoonful of the creamy coffee mixture on the top of each glass and stir before serving.

Keto Eggnog

Servings: 4

Time: 10 mins

Difficulty: Easy

Nutrients per serving: Calories: 249 kcal | Fat: 24g | Carbohydrates: 6g | Protein: 3g | Fiber: 1g

Ingredients

- 1/4 Cup Orange Juice
- 2 Egg Yolks
- 1/2 Tbsp. Orange Zest
- 1/4 Tbsp. Vanilla
- 1/2 Tsp. Erythritol, Powdered
- 1/8 Tsp. Nutmeg, Ground
- 1 Cup Heavy Whipping Cream
- 4 Tbsps. Bourbon Or Brandy (Optional)

Method

1. Combine egg yolks, vanilla extract, and erythritol in a deep bowl and whisk the mixture well until it becomes fluffy.
2. Add in the orange juice, orange zest, and whipping cream. Mix well until a smooth consistency is attained.
3. Pour the eggnog n the serving glasses and refrigerate for about 15 minutes.
4. Finally, serve with a sprinkle of nutmeg on top.

Iced Tea

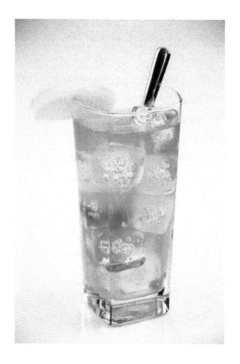

Servings: 2

Time: 2 hrs. & 10 mins

Difficulty: Easy

Nutrients per serving: Calories: 0 kcal | Fat: 0g | Carbohydrates: 0g | Protein: 0g | Fiber: 0g

Ingredients

- 1 Tea Bag
- 2 Cups Cold Water
- 1 Cup Ice Cubes
- 1/3 Cup Sliced Lemon or Fresh Mint Leaves

Method

1. Put the teabag and lemon slices or mint leaves in a cup of cold water in a pitcher and put in the refrigerator for an hour or two.
2. Take the tea bag, and lemon slices or mint leaves out of the water. Substitute them with new ones if you want.
3. Pour in another cup of water and ice cubes in the pitcher and serve.

Flavored Water

Servings: 4

Time: 5 mins

Difficulty: Easy

Nutrients per serving: Calories: 0 kcal | Fat: 0g | Carbohydrates: 0g | Protein: 0g | Fiber: 0g

Ingredients

- 2 Cups Ice Cubes
- Flavoring, e.g., Fresh Mint Or Raspberries, Or Sliced Cucumber
- 4 Cups Cold Water

Method

1. Take a pitcher and add cold water along with flavorings in it.
2. Refrigerate it for about 30 minutes and then serve.

Butter Coffee

Servings: 1

Time: 5 mins

Difficulty: Easy

Nutrients per serving: Calories: 0 kcal | Fat: 37g | Carbohydrates: 0g | Protein: 1g | Fiber: 0g

Ingredients

- 2 Tbsps. Butter, Unsalted
- 1 Tbsp. Coconut Or MCT Oil
- 1 Cup Freshly Brewed Coffee, Hot

Method

1. Brew your coffee according to your preference, and let it cool down a bit.
2. Combine the coffee with all the other ingredients in a blender and blend for about a minute or until it becomes frothy.
3. Pour the butter coffee in your favorite mug and enjoy.

Keto Hot Chocolate

Servings: 1

Time: 5 mins

Difficulty: Easy

Nutrients per serving: Calories: 216 kcal | Fat: 23g | Carbohydrates: 1g | Protein: 1g | Fiber: 2g

Ingredients

- 1 Cup Boiling Water
- 2 & 1/2 Tsps. Powdered Erythritol
- 2 Tbsps. Butter, Unsalted
- 1/4 Tsp. Vanilla Extract
- 1 Tbsp. Cocoa Powder

Method

1. Combine all the ingredients in a full-sized mug and blend well with an immersion blender until it becomes frothy.
2. Serve hot and enjoy.

Dairy-Free Keto Latte

Servings: 2

Time: 5 mins

Difficulty: Easy

Nutrients per serving: Calories: 191 kcal | Fat: 18g | Carbohydrates: 1g | Protein: 6g | Fiber: 0g

Ingredients

- 1 & 1/2 Cups Boiling Water
- 2 Tbsps. Coconut Oil
- 1 Tsp. Ground Ginger Or Pumpkin Pie Spice
- 2 Eggs
- 1/8 Tsp. Vanilla Extract

Method

1. Combine all the ingredients in a blender and blend for a few seconds.
2. Do not let the eggs cook in the boiling water and serve instantly.

Low-Carb Vegan Vanilla Protein Shake

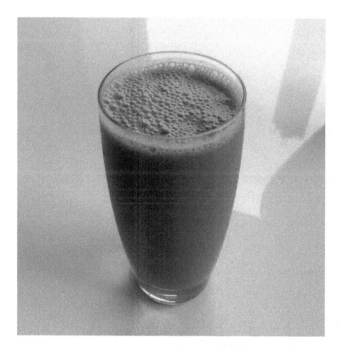

Servings: 1

Time: 10 mins

Difficulty: Easy

Nutrients per serving: Calories: 449 kcal | Fat: 34g | Carbohydrates: 8g | Protein: 28g | Fiber: 4g

Ingredients

- 4 Tbsps. Pea Protein Powder, Unflavored
- 1/2 Cup Almond Milk, Unsweetened
- 2 Tbsps. Cauliflower Rice, Frozen
- 1 Tbsp. Almond Butter
- 1/2 Cup Coconut Milk
- 1 Tsp. Vanilla Extract
- 1/2 Tsp. Cinnamon, Ground

Method

1. Combine all the ingredients in a blender and blend the mixture for a minute or until a smooth consistency is attained.
2. Decant in a serving glass and enjoy.

Electrolyte Elixir

Servings: 4

Time: 1 min

Difficulty: Easy

Nutrients per serving: Calories: 7 kcal | Fat: 0.1g | Carbohydrates: 2g | Protein: 0.1g | Fiber: 0g

Ingredients

- 1/2 Cup Lemon Juice, Fresh
- 1/2 Tsp. Magnesium
- 1 Tsp. Salt
- 8 Cups Water

Method

1. Combine all the ingredients in a pitcher and stir well.
2. Decant in serving glasses and enjoy.

Keto Chai Latte

Servings: 2

Time: 5 mins

Difficulty: Beginner

Nutrients per serving: Calories: 133 kcal | Fat: 14g | Carbohydrates: 1g | Protein: 1g | Fiber: 0g

Ingredients

- 2 Cups Boiling Water
- 1/3 Cup Heavy Whipping Cream
- 1 Tbsp. Chai Tea

Method

1. According to the package instructions, brew the tea in boiling water.
2. In a saucepan or microwave, heat the cream and pour it into the tea and serve.

Sugar-Free Mulled Wine

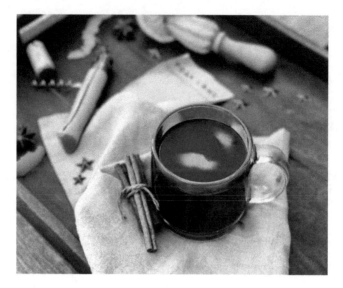

Servings: 8

Time: 15 mins

Difficulty: Beginner

Nutrients per serving: Calories: 82 kcal | Fat: 0.1g | Carbohydrates: 3g | Protein: 0.1g | Fiber: 0g

Ingredients

- 2 Cinnamon Sticks

- 1 & 1/2 Tsps. Orange Zest, Dried
- 1 Star Anise
- 2 Tsps. Ginger, Dried
- 1 Tsp. Green Cardamom Seeds
- 3 Cups White Or Red Wine, With Or Without Alcohol
- 1 Tsp. Cloves
- 1 Tbsp. Vanilla Extract (Optional)

Method

1. Combine all the ingredients in a saucepan and simmer over medium-low flame for about 5-10 minutes. Do not bring to boil.
2. Remove from the heat and let the mixture sit overnight for a strong taste of spices.
3. Strain the wine and serve hot with snacks or nuts.

Co-Keto (Puerto Rican Coconut Eggnog)

Servings: 2

Time: 5 mins

Difficulty: Easy

Nutrients per serving: Calories: 563kcal | Fat: 56g| Carbohydrates: 7g | Protein: 7g| Fiber: 0g

Ingredients

- 3 & 1/3 Cups Coconut Cream
- 2 Cups Heavy Whipping Cream
- 4 Egg Yolks, Beaten
- 1 & 2/3 Cups Coconut Milk, Unsweetened
- 1 Cup Rum
- 1/2 Cup Warm Water
- 2 Tbsps. Coconut Oil
- 1 Tbsp. Vanilla Extract
- Stevia, To Taste
- 2 Tsps. Cinnamon, Ground
- 1/4 Tsp. Ginger, Ground
- 1/4 Tsp. Nutmeg, Ground
- 1/4 Tsp. Cloves, Ground

Method

1. Heat the beaten egg yolks and whipping cream together in a double boiler, constantly stirring until a smooth consistency is attained and the temperature reaches 160°F.
2. Add the coconut oil and mix well until thick and smooth.
3. Pour this mixture into a blender and add all the other ingredients. Blend well and then transfer to the glass bottles and let chill.

Cinnamon Coffee

Servings: 1

Time: 5 mins

Difficulty: Easy

Nutrients per serving: Calories: 660 kcal | Fat: 60g | Carbohydrates: 7g | Protein: 13g | Fiber: 7g

Ingredients

- 1/2 Tsp. Brown Sugar
- 1/8 Tsp. Cinnamon, Powdered
- Whipped Cream (Optional)
- 1 Cup Coffee

Method

1. According to the package instructions, brew the coffee.
2. Add the brown sugar and cinnamon powder to it and stir well.
3. Put a dollop of whipped cream on top if you want.

Sugar-Free Caramel Brulee Latte

Servings: 2

Time: 2 mins

Difficulty: Easy

Nutrients per serving: Calories: 106 kcal | Fat: 11g | Carbohydrates: 1g | Protein: 1g |

Ingredients

- 2 Tbsps. Caramel Syrup
- 2 Cups Brewed Coffee
- 4 Tbsps. Coconut Milk Or Heavy Whipped Cream

Method

1. Brew your coffee according to your preference and add one Tbsp. of caramel syrup and 2 Tbsps. of coconut milk or heavy cream in each cup.
2. Top with a dollop of whipped cream or caramel if you want and serve.

Pumpkin Spice Latte Milkshakes

Servings: 3

Time: 15 mins

Difficulty: Easy

Nutrients per serving (with 2 Tbsps. whipped coconut cream per shake): Calories: 364 kcal | Fat: 18.52g| Carbohydrates: 5.48g | Protein: 2.3g| Fiber: 1.83g

Ingredients

- 1 Cup Keto Vanilla Ice Cream
- 1/3 Cup Almond Milk
- 1/3 Cup Water
- 2 Tbsps. Pumpkin Puree
- 1 & 1/2 Tsp. Instant Coffee
- 1 Tsp. Pumpkin Pie Spice

Coconut Whipped Cream:
- 2 Tbsps. Sugar (Low Carb)
- 1 & 3/4 Cups Coconut Milk

Method

1. Put the coconut milk in the refrigerator overnight, take the thick cream off the milk top, and put it in a bowl. Save the milk for other recipes.
2. Whisk in the low carb sugar in the coconut cream until your desired consistency is attained.
3. Combine all the other ingredients in a blender and blend for a few minutes until it becomes smooth.
4. Decant in your preferred glasses and top with coconut whipped cream.

Keto Russian Coffee

Servings: 2

Time: 2 mins

Difficulty: Easy

Nutrients per serving: Calories: 214 kcal | Fat: 22g | Carbohydrates: 3g | Protein: 2g | Fiber: 1g

Ingredients

- 1/3 Cup Vanilla Vodka
- 4 Tbsps. Almond Milk, Unsweetened
- 2 Tbsps. Stevia
- 2 Cups Brewed Coffee

Milk Foam (Optional)
- 1/4 Cup Heavy Cream
- 2 Tbsps. French Vanilla Whipped Foam Topping (Sugar-Free)
- 1 Stick Of Cinnamon
- 1/4 Tsp. Vanilla Extract

Method

1. Brew coffee according to your preference and divide it into two cups. Stir in half of the almond milk, Stevia, and vodka in each cup.
2. Put the milk foam on top if you want.
3. To make milk foam, combine all its ingredients in a jar and mix well until the mixture becomes frothy. Microwave for 10 sec and then put a dollop on each serving.

Creamy Matcha Latte

Servings: 1

Time: 6 mins

Difficulty: Easy

Nutrients per serving: Calories: 255 kcal | Fat: 22.8g| Carbohydrates: 5.3g | Protein: 2.33g | Fiber: 1.3g

Ingredients

- 1/8 Tsp. Pink Sea Salt
- 1/3 Cup Almond Milk, Unsweetened
- 1 Tsp. Matcha Tea
- 2/3 Cup Coconut Milk
- Stevia, To Taste
- 4 Drops Vanilla Extract (Optional)

Method

1. Take a saucepan and add both kinds of milk to it. Heat until it starts to bubble and add the remaining ingredients to it.
2. Mix well and serve in separate cups.

Keto Avocado Smoothie

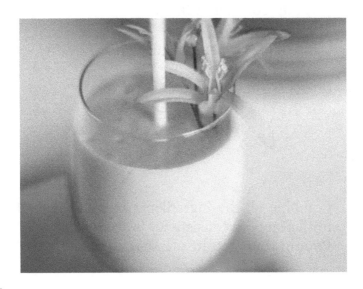

Servings: 2

Time: 10 mins

Difficulty: Easy

Nutrients per serving: Calories: 232 kcal | Fat: 22.4g | Carbohydrates: 6.9g | Protein: 1.7g | Fiber: 2.8g

Ingredients

- 1/2 Tsp. Turmeric Powder

- 1 Tsp. Fresh Ginger, Grated
- 1/4 Cup Almond Milk
- 3/4 Cup Coconut Milk
- 1/2 Avocado
- 1 Tsp. Lime Or Lemon Juice
- 1 Cup Ice, Crushed
- Stevia, To Taste

Method

1. Combine all the ingredients in a blender and blend until a smooth consistency is attained.
2. Pour in your favorite glasses and enjoy.

Avocado Mint Green Keto Smoothie

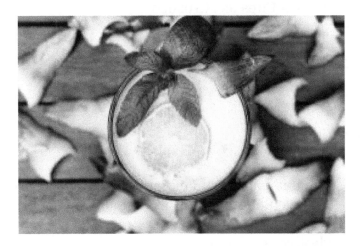

Servings: 1

Time: 2 mins

Difficulty: Easy

Nutrients per serving: Calories: 223 kcal | Fat: 23g | Carbohydrates: 5g | Protein: 1g | Fiber: 1g

Ingredients

- 1/2 Cup Almond Milk
- 5-6 Mint Leaves
- 1/2 Avocado

- 3/4 Cup Coconut Milk
- 1/2 Tsp. Lime Juice
- 1 & 1/2 Cups Ice, Crushed
- Stevia, To Taste
- 3 Cilantro Sprigs
- 1/4 Tsp. Vanilla Extract

Method

1. Combine all the ingredients in a blender, except ice, and blend until it becomes smooth.
2. Then, add the crushed ice and blend again till the desired consistency.
3. Pour into glasses and serve.

Keto Skinny Margaritas

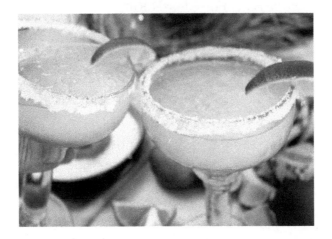

Servings: 2

Time: 10 mins

Difficulty: Easy

Nutrients per serving: Calories: 102 kcal | Fat: 1g | Carbohydrates: 1g | Protein: 1g

Ingredients

- 1/3 Cup Tequila
- 1 Tbsp. Warm Water
- 2 Tbsps. Lime Juice

- Ice Cubes, To Taste
- Stevia, To Taste
- Coarse Salt, For Glass's Rim

Method

1. Mix the warm water and Stevia in a bowl and put squeeze the lime juice in another bowl.
2. Take a jar and combine the lime juice, sweetener syrup, and the tequila in it. Close the lid of the jar and shake it well to mix the contents.
3. Slightly wet the rim of two cocktail glasses and line with salt, and pour the margarita in them.
4. Add the ice in them and garnish with a slice of fresh lime if you want.

Iced Keto Matcha Green Tea Latte

Servings: 1

Time: 1 min

Difficulty: Easy

Nutrients per serving: Calories: 36 kcal | Fat: 2.5g | Carbohydrates: 0.8g | Protein: 1.6g | Fiber: 0.8g

Ingredients

- 5 Drops Vanilla Stevia
- 1 Tsp. Matcha Powder
- 1 Cup Coconut Or Vanilla Almond Milk, Unsweetened
- Ice, To Taste

Method

1. Combine all ingredients in a blender and blend for a few minutes until a smooth consistency is attained and match if completely dissolved.
2. Add ice in your preferred quantity and enjoy.

Spiced Gingerbread Coffee

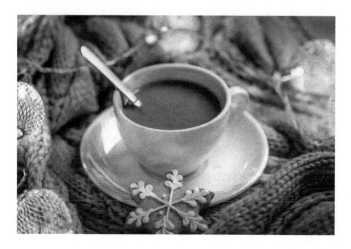

Servings: 1

Time: 2 mins

Difficulty: Easy

Nutrients per serving: Calories: 108 kcal | Fat: 11.2g | Carbohydrates: 1.5g | Protein: 1g

Ingredients

- 1 Cup Hot Brewed Coffee
- 1 Tbsp. Heavy Cream
- 1/2 Tsp. Sukrin Gold

- 1 & 1/2 Tsps. Sukrin Gold Fiber Syrup
- 1/4 Tsp. Ginger, Ground
- 1/8 Tsp. Cloves, Ground
- 1/8 Tsp. Cinnamon, Ground
- Whipped Cream

Method

1. Combine all the ingredients in a mug except cloves and cream. Mix well until the spices are blended thoroughly.
2. Add a dollop of whipped cream on top and sprinkle the ground cloves on it.

Coconut Milk Strawberry Smoothie

Servings: 2

Time: 2 mins

Difficulty: Easy

Nutrients per serving: Calories: 397 kcal | Fat: 37g | Carbohydrates: 15g | Protein: 6g | Fiber: 5g

Ingredients

- 2 Tbsps. Almond Butter, Smooth
- 1 Cup Coconut Milk, Unsweetened
- 3/4 Tsp. Stevia (Optional)
- 1 Cup Strawberries, Frozen

Method

1. Combine all the ingredients in a blender and mix until a smooth consistency is attained.
2. Decant into the serving glasses and enjoy.

Peanut Butter Chocolate Keto Milkshake

Servings: 1

Time: 1 min

Difficulty: Easy

Nutrients per serving: Calories: 79 kcal | Fat: 5.7g | Carbohydrates: 6.4g | Protein: 3.6g | Fiber: 3.3g

Ingredients

- 5 Drops Stevia
- 1/8 Tsp. Sea Salt
- 1 Tbsp. Peanut Butter Powder, Unsweetened
- 1 Cup Coconut Milk, Unsweetened
- 1 Tbsp. Cocoa Powder, Unsweetened

Method

1. Combine all the ingredients in a blender and mix until a smooth consistency is attained.
2. Decant into the serving glasses and enjoy.

Sugar-Free Fresh Squeezed Lemonade

Servings: 8

Time: 10 mins

Difficulty: Easy

Nutrients per serving: Calories: 5 kcal | Fat: 1g | Carbohydrates: 2g | Protein: 1g | Fiber: 1g

Ingredients

- 8 Cups Water
- 1 Tsp. Lemon Monkfruit Drops
- 4 Slices Lemon (Optional)
- 3/4 Cup Lemon Juice
- Ice (Optional)

Method

1. Combine all the ingredients in a pitcher and stir well to mix.
2. Chill in the refrigerator or add ice to it before serving.
3. Put the lemon slices in it if you want.

Cucumber Mint Water

Servings: 16

Time: 5 mins

Difficulty: Easy

Nutrients per serving: Calories: 3 kcal | Fat: 0g | Carbohydrates: 0g | Protein: 0g | Fiber: 0g

Ingredients

- 8 Cups Water
- 3/4 Cup Cucumber Slices
- 1 Tbsps. Mint Leaves

Method

1. Press the mint leaves in a pitcher with the help of a spoon and add the other ingredients to it.
2. Chill it in the refrigerator for an hour and then enjoy.

Caramel Apple Drink

Servings: 1

Time: 10 mins

Difficulty: Easy

Nutrients per serving: Calories: 76 kcal | Fat: 3g | Carbohydrates: 16g | Protein: 1g | Fiber: 14g

Ingredients

- 2 Cups Water
- 1 Tbsp. Caramel Syrup
- 1 Tbsp. Apple Cider Vinegar (Raw)
- 1/8 Tsp. Allspice
- 1/8 Tsp. Nutmeg, Ground
- 1/8 Tsp. Orange Zest, Dried
- 1 Cinnamon Stick, Halved
- 3 Whole Cloves
- 1/4 Cup Vanilla Whipped Cream (Optional)
- 1/8 Tsp. Cinnamon, Ground (Optional)
- 5 Drops Stevia (Optional)

Method

1. Take the water in a pan and put the allspice, cinnamon stick halves, and cloves in it. Boil the water and then let it sit for 2-3 minutes off the heat, with the lid on.
2. Strain the spice water into a large mug and put the caramel syrup and apple cider vinegar in it. Stir well and add Stevia or ground cinnamon if you want.
3. Put a dollop of whipped cream on top if you ant and drizzle some caramel syrup if you want.

Keto Frosty Chocolate Shake

Servings: 1

Time: 10 mins

Difficulty: Easy

Nutrients per serving: Calories: 346 kcal | Fat: 36g | Carbohydrates: 8.4g | Protein: 4g | Fiber: 4g

Ingredients

- 5 Tbsps. Almond Milk, Unsweetened
- 2 Tbsps. Cocoa Powder
- 1 & 1/2 Tsps. Truvia
- 1/8 Tsp. Vanilla Extract (Sugar-Free)
- 6 Tbsps. Heavy Whipping Cream

Method

1. Combine all the ingredients and whisk well to make a fluffy peak of cream.
2. Freeze the mixture for 20 minutes and then crack it open with a fork.
3. Chill it as per your preference and serve cold.

Strawberry Avocado Smoothie

Servings: 2

Time: 2 mins

Difficulty: Easy

Nutrients per serving: Calories: 165 kcal | Fat: 14g| Carbohydrates: 11g | Protein: 2g | Fiber: 7g

Ingredients

- 1 & 1/2 Cups Coconut Milk
- 1 Tsp. Stevia
- 1 Avocado
- 1 Tbsp. Lime Juice
- 2/3 Cup Strawberries, Frozen
- 1/2 Cup Ice

Method

1. Combine all the ingredients in a blender and blend until a smooth consistency is attained.
2. Pour in your favorite glasses and enjoy.

Almond Berry Mini Cheesecake Smoothies

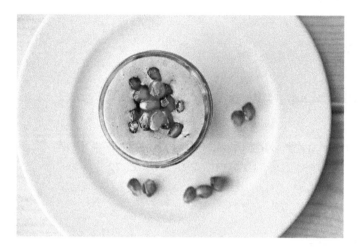

Servings: 2

Time: 10 mins

Difficulty: Easy

Nutrients per serving: Calories: 165 kcal | Fat: 8.6g | Carbohydrates: 16.8g | Protein: 7g | Fiber: 4.4g

Ingredients

- 1 Cup Almond Or Coconut Milk, Chilled

- 2 Tbsps. Almond Or Coconut Flour
- 2 Cups Mixed Berries, Frozen
- 1 Tbsp. Almond Butter, Smooth
- 1/2 Cup Cottage Cheese, Organic
- 1 Tsp. Nuts Or Almonds, Toasted & Crushed
- 1 Tsp. Vanilla Extract
- 1/8 Tsp. Cinnamon
- Stevia, To Taste (Optional)

Method

1. Combine all the ingredients in a blender, except crushed nuts, and blend until a smooth consistency is attained.
2. You can add Stevia if you want and pour it into cups.
3. Top with crushed and toasted nuts and serve.

Hemp Milk And Nut Milk

Servings: 4

Time: 12 hrs. 15 mins

Difficulty: Easy

Nutrients per serving: Calories: 44 kcal | Fat: 3.6g | Carbohydrates: 1.7g | Protein: 1.5g | Fiber: 0.9g

Ingredients

Nut milk

- 4 Cups Water
- 1/8 Tsp. Sea Salt
- 1 Cup Raw Nuts (Pecan, Almond, Walnut, Cashew, etc.)
- 1 Tsp. Vanilla Extract (Optional)
- 1/3 Cup Maple Syrup (Optional)

For Hemp Milk

- 3 Cups Water
- 1/8 Tsp. Sea Salt
- 1/2 Cup Hulled Hemp Seed
- 1/4 Cup Maple Syrup (Optional)
- 1 Tsp. Vanilla Extract (Optional)

Method

Nut Milk

1. Soak the nuts overnight and drain them the next day.
2. Blend the water and soaked nuts in a blender until a smooth consistency is attained.
3. Add in the salt, vanilla extract, and maple syrup if you want and blend again until mixed well.
4. Strain the mixture using a double layer of cheesecloth to isolate the pulp. Once done, add water to the milk to get your preferred consistency.
5. Pour the nut milk into mason jars and store them if you want for up to 5 days.
6. Cover the jars with lids and store in the refrigerator for up to 5 days.

Hemp Milk

1. Combine all the ingredients in a blender and blend for a few minutes or until a smooth consistency is attained.
2. You can strain the excess seeds using a cheesecloth and store the hemp milk in mason jars for up to 5 days.

Gut Healing Bone Broth Latte

Servings: 2

Time: 10 mins

Difficulty: Easy

Nutrients per serving: Calories: 161 kcal | Fat: 7.2g | Carbohydrates: 5.2g | Protein: 10.8g | Fiber: 0.9g

Ingredients

- 1 Tbsp. Coconut Oil
- 1/4 Tsp. Ginger, Ground
- 2 Cups Bone Broth
- 1/8 Tsp. Cayenne Pepper
- 1/8 Tsp. Turmeric Powder
- 1/8 Tsp. Black Pepper
- 1/8 Tsp. Sea Salt
- Coconut Cream, To Taste (Optional)
- Collagen Peptides (Optional)

Savory Latte Toppings (Optional)
- Fresh Herbs
- Green Onion, Chopped
- Red Pepper Flakes

Method

1. Pour bone broth into a saucepan and add all the ingredients in it except sea salt.
2. Heat the mixture over medium flame while stirring constantly until combined.
3. You can use an immersion blender to mix coconut cream if necessary.
4. Blend well to make a frothy and creamy mixture.
5. Pour into serving mugs and sprinkle seal salt on top.
6. You can also use savory latte toppings for garnishing if you want.

Creamy Cocoa Coconut Low Carb Shake

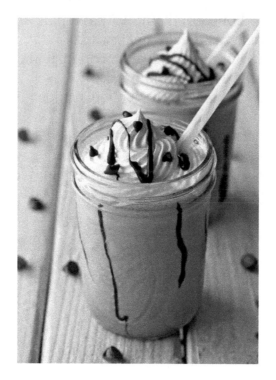

Servings: 2

Time: 5 mins

Difficulty: Easy

Nutrients per serving: Calories: 222 kcal | Fat: 23.1g | Carbohydrates: 5.4g | Protein: 2.5g | Fiber: 2.7g

Ingredients

- 2 Tbsps. Cocoa Powder
- 1/2 Tbsp. Almond Butter, Smooth
- 1 Cup Almond Or Coconut Milk, Unsweetened
- 2 Tbsps. Coconut MCT Oil
- 1/8 Tsp. Sea Salt
- 1/2 Cup Coconut Cream

Additional Sweeteners (Optional)

- Stevia Leaf Or Xylitol
- Banana Or Maple Syrup
- Cinnamon
- Berries

Method

1. Combine all the ingredients in a blender and mix until a smooth consistency is attained.
2. Add sweetener of your choice, if you want, and decant into the serving glasses and enjoy.

Low Carb Dark Chocolate Protein Smoothie

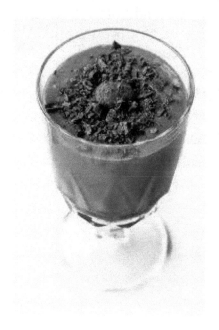

Servings: 1

Time: 5 mins

Difficulty: Easy

Nutrients per serving: Calories: 220 kcal | Fat: 9g | Carbohydrates: 2.5g | Protein: 28.4g | Fiber: 19.5g

Ingredients

- 1 Cup Almond Milk, Unsweetened
- 1/4 Cup Avocado, Frozen
- 1/2 Tsp. Matcha Green Tea
- 2 Tbsps. Protein Powder, Zero Carb
- 1 Tbsp. Swerve Sweetener
- 1 Tbsp. Cocoa Powder, Dark

Method

1. Combine all the ingredients in a blender and mix until a smooth consistency is attained.
2. Decant into the serving glass and enjoy.

Mint Chocolate Green Smoothie

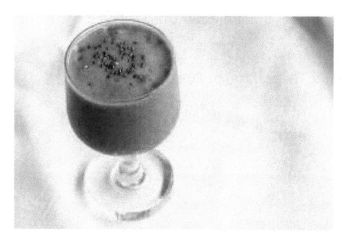

Servings: 2

Time: 5 mins

Difficulty: Easy

Nutrients per serving: Calories: 359 kcal | Fat: 17.4g | Carbohydrates: 37.4g | Protein: 20.6g | Fiber: 10g

Ingredients

- 3/4 Cup Vanilla Almond Milk, Unsweetened
- 1/2 Cup Ice
- 1/2 Cup Kale, Packed Firmly

- 1/4 Cup Vanilla Protein Powder
- 1/4 Cup Vanilla Greek Yogurt (2%)
- 1/4 Cup Avocado, Mashed
- 1 Tbsp. Mini Chocolate Chips
- 1/4 Tsp. Peppermint Extract
- 1/2 Tbsp. Agave

Method

1. Combine all the ingredients in a blender and mix until a smooth consistency is attained.
2. Decant into the serving glasses and enjoy.

Low Carb Raspberry Cheesecake Shake

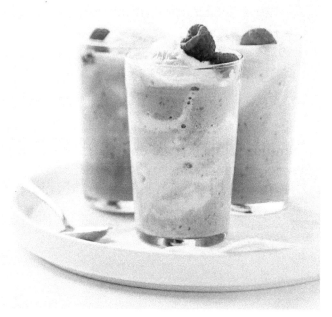

Servings: 1

Time: 5 mins

Difficulty: Easy

Nutrients per serving: Calories: 560 kcal | Fat: 55g | Carbohydrates: 8g | Protein: 9g | Fiber: 3g

Ingredients

- 1/4 Cup Almond Milk, Unsweetened
- 1 Tsp. Butter, Unsalted (Cold)
- 1/4 Cup Heavy Cream
- 6-8 Raspberries, Fresh
- 1/4 Cup Cream Cheese
- 4 Tsps. Almond Flour
- Ice (Optional)
- Liquid Stevia, To Taste (Optional)

Method

1. Put the almond milk, raspberries, heavy cream, and cream cheese in a vessel and blend using an immersion blender. Add the sweetener if you want. Transfer it into a serving glass.
2. In a bowl, mix the almond flour and butter to form crumbs. Put these crumbs on top of the drink after adding ice, if you want, and serve.

Watermelon Smoothie

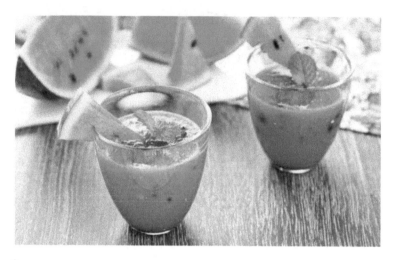

Servings: 1

Time: 5 mins

Difficulty: Easy

Nutrients per serving: Calories: 39 kcal | Fat: 3g | Carbohydrates: 1g | Protein: 0g

Ingredients

- 3/4 Cup Lemon Lime Seltzer
- 1/8 Tsp. Xantham Gum

- 15 Drops Watermelon Flavoring Oil
- 8 Ice Cubes
- 1 Drop Vanilla Extract
- 2 Tbsps. Stevia
- 1 Drop Lemon Extract
- 1. Tbsp Heavy Cream

Method

1. Combine all the ingredients in a blender and mix until a smooth consistency is attained.
2. Decant into the serving glass and enjoy.

Low-Carb Blueberry Smoothie

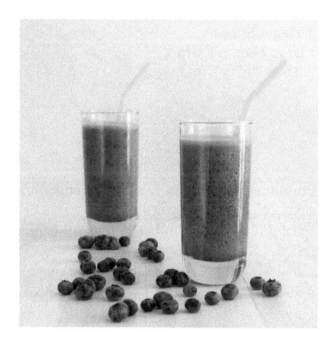

Servings: 2

Time: 5 mins

Difficulty: Easy

Nutrients per serving: Calories: 251 kcal | Fat: 22g | Carbohydrates: 6g | Protein: 8g | Fiber: 1g

Ingredients

- 1/4 Cup Cream Cheese
- 3/4 Cup Almond Milk, Unsweetened
- 1/2 Tsp. Vanilla Extract
- 1/2 Cup Ice
- 2 Tsps. Stevia/Erythritol Blend, Granulated
- 1/3 Cup Blueberries, Frozen
- 1-5 Drops Lemon Extract
- 1/4 Cup Heavy Whipping Cream
- 2 Tbsps. Collagen Peptides (Optional)

Method

1. Combine all the ingredients in a blender and mix until a smooth consistency is attained.
2. Decant into the serving glasses and enjoy.

Pumpkin Low Carb Smoothie With Salted Caramel

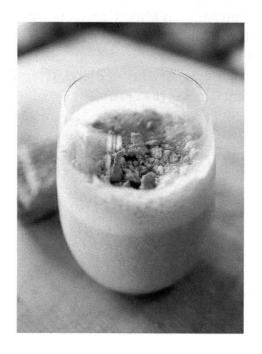

Servings: 1

Time: 5 mins

Difficulty: Easy

Nutrients per serving: Calories: 245 kcal | Fat: 10.4g | Carbohydrates: 11.8g | Protein: 29g | Fiber: 6.4g

Ingredients

- 1 Cup Almond Milk
- 1/4 Avocado
- 2 Tbsps. Vanilla Protein Powder
- 1/4 Cup Pumpkin Puree
- 4 Ice Cubes
- 2 Tbsps. Caramel Syrup, Salted & Sugar-Free

Method

1. Combine all the ingredients in a blender and mix until a smooth consistency is attained.
2. Decant into the serving glass and enjoy.

McKeto Strawberry Milkshake

Servings: 1

Time: 5 mins

Difficulty: Easy

Nutrients per serving: Calories: 368 kcal | Fat: 38.85g | Carbohydrates: 2.42g | Protein: 1.69g | Fiber: 1.28g

Ingredients

- 1/4 Cup Heavy Cream
- 1/4 Tsp. Xanthan Gum
- 3/4 Cup Coconut Milk
- 7 Ice Cubes
- 1 Tbsp. MCT Oil
- 2 Tbsps. Strawberry Torani, Sugar-Free

Method

1. Combine all the ingredients in a blender and mix until a smooth consistency is attained.
2. Decant into the serving glass and enjoy.

Keto Blueberry Cheesecake Smoothie

Servings: 1

Time: 5 mins

Difficulty: Easy

Nutrients per serving: Calories: 311 kcal | Fat: 27g | Carbohydrates: 9g | Protein: 5.5g | Fiber: 2.5g

Ingredients

- 1/2 Cup Cream Cheese
- 2 Tbsps. Heavy Cream
- 1 Cup Almond Milk, Unsweetened
- 1 Tsp. Cinnamon, Ground
- 1/2 Cup Blueberries
- 6 Drops Stevia
- 1/2 Tsp. Vanilla Extract

Method

1. Combine all the ingredients in a blender and mix until a smooth consistency is attained.
2. Decant into the serving glass and enjoy.

Keto Tropical Smoothie

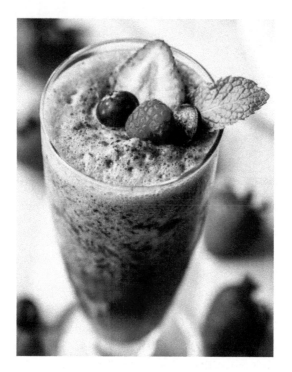

Servings: 2

Time: 5 mins

Difficulty: Easy

Nutrients per serving: Calories: 355.75 kcal | Fat: 32.63g | Carbohydrates: 4.41g | Protein: 4.4g | Fiber: 3g

Ingredients

- 1 Tbsp. MCT Oil
- 1/2 Tsp. Mango Extract
- 7 Ice Cubes
- 2 Tbsps. Golden Flaxseed Meal
- 1/4 Tsp. Blueberry Extract
- 3/4 Cup Coconut Milk, Unsweetened
- 1/4 Tsp. Banana Extract
- 1/4 Cup Sour Cream
- 20 Drops Liquid Stevia

Method

1. Combine all the ingredients in a blender and mix until a smooth consistency is attained. Let it sit for a few minutes and allow the flax meal to absorb moisture.
2. Decant into the serving glasses and enjoy.

Keto Kale & Coconut Shake

Servings: 1

Time: 5 mins

Difficulty: Easy

Nutrients per serving: Calories: 660 kcal | Fat: 60g | Carbohydrates: 7g | Protein: 13g | Fiber: 7g

Ingredients

- 4 Cups Kale, Chopped
- 1/2 Cup Coconut Milk
- 1 Cup Almond Milk, Unsweetened
- 1/4 Cup Coconut, Unsweetened & Ground
- 1 Cup Ice
- 1/4 Tsp. Kosher Salt
- 1 Tbsp. Fresh Ginger, Peeled (Optional)

Method

1. Combine all the ingredients in a blender and mix until a smooth consistency is attained.
2. Decant into the serving glass and enjoy.

Savory Cucumber Herb Sangria

Servings: 2-4

Time: 5 mins

Difficulty: Easy

Nutrients per serving: Calories: 660 kcal | Fat: 60g | Carbohydrates: 7g | Protein: 13g | Fiber: 7g

Ingredients

- 2 Cups Sparkling Water
- 3 Cups Dry White Wine
- 2 Cups Ice
- 3 Limes, Sliced
- 1 Green Cucumber, Sliced
- 1 Cup Basil Leaves, Fresh
- 2 Lemons, Sliced
- 1 Cup Mint Leaves, Fresh

Method

1. Put all ingredients in a pitcher except wine, sparkling water, and ice. Stir well and press the lemon, lime,

basil, mint, and cucumber a little to release their juices.
2. Add the wine to it and stir well.
3. Put it in the refrigerator and let it sit for about 20 minutes.
4. Take out the pitcher and pour in the sparkling water and ice.
5. Serve cold.

Sparkling Raspberry Limeade Mocktail

Servings: 2

Time: 1 min

Difficulty: Easy

Nutrients per serving: Calories: 22 kcal | Fat: 0.2g | Carbohydrates: 5.5g | Protein: 0.5g | Fiber: 2.1g

Ingredients

- 1/2 Cup Raspberries, Unsweetened & Frozen
- 1 & 1/2 Cups Sparkling Raspberry Lemonade, Chilled
- 2 Tbsps. Lime Juice
- 1/8 Tsp. Vanilla Stevia
- 1/2 Cup Ice, Crushed

Method

1. Combine all the ingredients in a blender and mix until a smooth consistency is attained.
2. Decant into the serving glasses and enjoy.

Bailey's Irish Cream

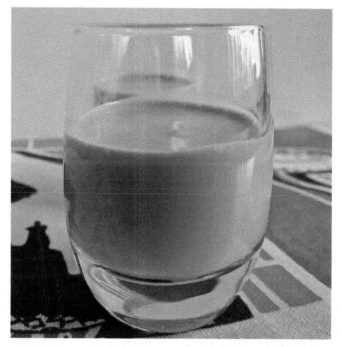

Servings: 12

Time: 20 mins

Difficulty: Easy

Nutrients per serving: Calories: 200 kcal | Fat: 14g | Carbohydrates: 1g | Protein: 0g | Fiber: 0g

Ingredients

- 1/2 Tsp. Vanilla Extract
- 1 & 1/4 Cups Irish Whiskey
- 2 Cups Heavy Cream
- 1 Tbsp. Cocoa Powder
- 1/2 Tsp. Instant Espresso Powder
- 2/3 Cup Swerve
- 1 Tsp. Almond Extract

Method

1. Take a saucepan and put cocoa, instant powder, sweetener, and cream in it. Heat it over medium-low flame and bring to a boil.
2. Reduce heat to low and let it simmer for about 10 minutes.
3. Take off the heat and add in the whiskey, almond, and vanilla extracts.
4. Let cool and serve.

Low Carb Coffee Milkshake

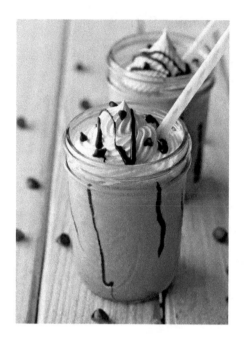

Servings: 2

Time: 1 min

Difficulty: Easy

Nutrients per serving: Calories: 345 kcal | Fat: 31.4g | Carbohydrates: 24g | Protein: 2.5g | Fiber: 18.2g

Ingredients

- 1 Tsp. Instant Espresso Powder
- 15 Drops Stevia
- 1 & 1/2 Cups Ice, Crushed
- 1 Cup Vanilla Ice Cream (Low Carb)
- 1/2 Cup Almond Milk
- 2 Tsps. Cocoa Powder (Optional)
- 2 Tbsps. Whipped Cream (Optional)

Method

1. Combine all the ingredients in a blender and mix until a smooth consistency is attained.
2. Decant into the serving glasses and put a dollop of whipped cream on top if you want.

Sugar-Free Strawberry Limeade

Servings: 8

Time: 5 mins

Difficulty: Easy

Nutrients per serving: Calories: 16 kcal | Fat: 0.1g | Carbohydrates: 4.3g | Protein: 0.2g | Fiber: 1.5g

Ingredients

- 5 Cups Water
- 3/4 Cup Lime Juice, Fresh
- 1 & 1/2 Tsps. Stevia
- 1 & 1/2 Cups Strawberries, Sliced
- Ice, To Taste

Method

1. Combine all the ingredients in a blender and mix until a smooth consistency is attained.
2. Decant into the serving glasses and enjoy.

Low-Carb Keto Shamrock Shake

Servings: 1

Time: 2 mins

Difficulty: Easy

Nutrients per serving: Calories: 660 kcal | Fat: 60g | Carbohydrates: 7g | Protein: 13g | Fiber: 7g

Ingredients

- 1 Tsp. Spinach Powder
- 1 Cup Vanilla Ice Cream, Low Carb
- 1/3 Cup Coconut Or Almond Milk, Unsweetened
- 1/8 Tsp. Pure Mint Extract
- Whipped Cream (Optional)

Method

1. Combine all the ingredients in a blender and mix until a smooth consistency is attained.
2. Decant into the serving glasses and put a dollop of whipped cream on top if you want.

Keto Smoothie With Almond Milk

Servings: 1

Time: 5 mins

Difficulty: Easy

Nutrients per serving: Calories: 332 kcal | Fat: 28.5g | Carbohydrates: 15g | Protein: 10.2g | Fiber: 8.9g

Ingredients

- 1 Tbsp. Cocoa Powder, Unsweetened
- 2 Tbsps. Almond Butter
- 1 Cup Almond Milk
- 1/4 Cup Avocado
- 3 Tbsps. Monkfruit
- 1 Cup Ice, Crushed

Method

1. Combine all the ingredients in a blender and mix until a smooth consistency is attained.
2. Decant into the serving glass and enjoy.

Sparkling Grapefruit Frosé

Servings: 6

Time: 5 mins

Difficulty: Easy

Nutrients per serving: Calories: 244 kcal | Fat: 0.1g | Carbohydrates: 29.1g | Protein: 1g | Fiber: 0.1g

Ingredients

- 1 Cup Ice
- 1 Cup Grapefruit Juice, Fresh
- 1/4 Cup Agave Nectar
- 1 & 1/2 Cups Rosé Wine

For Garnish (Optional)
- Grapefruit Wedges
- Mint Sprigs

Method

1. Freeze rosé in a shallow dish overnight.

2. Scrape it off the dish the next day and put in a blender with all other ingredients.
3. Blend until a smooth consistency is attained.
4. Decant into the serving glasses and garnish with mint sprigs and grapefruit wedges if you want.

Banana Oat Breakfast Smoothie

Servings: 2

Time: 5 mins

Difficulty: Easy

Nutrients per serving: Calories: 210 kcal | Fat: 7.5g | Carbohydrates: 32.5g | Protein: 5.6g | Fiber: 4.8g

Ingredients

- 1 Banana
- 1/2 Cup Almond Milk
- 1 Tbsp. Flaxseed Meal
- 1/2 Cup Yogurt
- 1/2 Tsp. Cinnamon
- 1/3 Cup Rolled Oats

Method

1. Combine all the ingredients in a blender and mix until a smooth consistency is attained.
2. Decant into the serving glasses and enjoy.

Keto Mexican Chocolate Eggnog

Servings: 6

Time: 15 mins

Difficulty: Easy

Nutrients per serving: Calories: 242 kcal | Fat: 23g | Carbohydrates: 4g | Protein: 7g | Fiber: 1g

Ingredients

- 1/4 Cup Whiskey Or Bourbon
- 1 & 1/2 Cups Almond Milk, Unsweetened
- 6 Eggs
- 1/4 Cup Cocoa Powder
- 1/2 Cup Monkfruit/Erythritol Blend
- 1 Cup Heavy Cream
- 1/2 Cup Whipped Cream
- 1 Tsp. Vanilla
- 1/2 Tsp. Cinnamon Powder
- 1/4 Tsp. Chili Powder
- 1/8 Tsp. Cayenne Pepper
- 1/8 Tsp. Nutmeg, Grated
- 1/8 Tsp. Salt

Method

1. Combine all the ingredients in a blender except bourbon/whiskey, vanilla, and whipped cream. Blend it until a smooth consistency is attained.
2. Then pour this mixture into a saucepan and heat it over a medium-low flame with constant stirring for about 8 minutes. Do not let it boil.
3. Take off the heat, put the saucepan in a bowl full of ice, and stir the eggnog to cool it down.
4. Add the bourbon/whiskey and vanilla in it and decant into a covered container.
5. Refrigerate for about 4 hours and add in the whipped cream or top the eggnog with it.
6. Serve and enjoy.

Keto Cranberry Hibiscus Margarita

Servings: 8

Time: 20 mins

Difficulty: Easy

Nutrients per serving: Calories: 86 kcal | Fat: 1g | Carbohydrates: 6g | Protein: 1g | Fiber: 2g

Ingredients

- 2 & 1/2 Tbsps. Naval Orange Zest
- 1 & 1/2 Cups Cranberries, Fresh
- 1 Cup Tequila
- 5 Cup Water
- 3/4 Cups + 2 Tbsps. Monkfruit/Erythritol Blend
- 3 Tbsps. Lime Juice, Fresh
- Ice
- 4 Hibiscus Tea Bags
- Coarse Salt, For Glass's Rim

Method

1. Take a saucepan and put the 1 cup water, 3/4 cup sweetener, orange zest, and cranberries in it. Heat it

over medium flame and bring to boil, reduce heat, and let it simmer until it is thickened, for about 10-15 minutes.

2. Strain the cranberry gel and let cool.
3. Boil the remaining 4 cups of water in a saucepan and put the hibiscus tea bags in it for five minutes.
4. Take out the tea bags and add the 2 Tbsps. of sweetener in it. Mix well and set aside to cool down.
5. Combine the cranberry gel, hibiscus tea, and all the remaining ingredients in a blender and blend well.
6. Slightly wet the rim of cocktail glasses and line with salt, and pour the margarita in them.

Keto Frozen Blackberry Lemonade

Servings: 2

Time: 5 mins

Difficulty: Easy

Nutrients per serving: Calories: 155 kcal | Fat: 15g | Carbohydrates: 6g | Protein: 2g | Fiber: 2g

Ingredients

- 1 Cup Ice
- 1/4 Cup Blackberries, Fresh
- 4 Tbsps. Lemon Juice
- 1/2 Cup Almond Milk
- 1/3 Cup Coconut Cream
- 1 Tbsp. Stevia/Erythritol Blend
- 1/8 Tsp. Sea Salt

Method

1. Combine all the ingredients in a blender and mix until a smooth consistency is attained.
2. Decant into the serving glasses and enjoy.

Lightning Source UK Ltd.
Milton Keynes UK
UKHW020419070521
383233UK00001BA/71